Bryan Dorsey, M.D

OUTSMART FAT FAST

A Definitive Guide to Burning Fat, Boost Energy and Balance Hormones

Table of Contents

This page was left blank intentionally

Preface

Betty, a mother of three in her forties, had battled weight issues for most of her existence. Nothing worked even though she had attempted every trendy diet and exercise regimen imaginable. Betty was on the verge of giving up when she discovered a novel method of weight reduction that would forever alter her outlook.

This strategy differed from another crash diet that promised quick weight reduction or a new exercise fad that would leave her worn out and irritated. Instead, it thoroughly explained how to balance hormones, grasp the science behind fat reduction, lose weight, and improve general health.

Experts in diet and exercise conducted years of study and testing to create this book, **"Outsmart Fat Fast: A Definitive Guide to Burning Fat, Boost Energy, and Balance Hormones."** It offers a thorough and simple-to-follow strategy that can assist anyone in achieving their weight reduction objectives while enhancing energy levels and general health.

The manual is not a one-size-fits-all solution or another fast remedy. Instead, it offers users individualized solutions that fit their specific requirements and way of life. This guide has something for everyone, whether you're a busy working mom like Betty or an exercise fanatic seeking to advance your weight reduction efforts.

"Outsmart Fat Fast" explains the science of diet, hormone homeostasis, and fat reduction in simple and understandable terms, making weight loss approachable and feasible for everyone. The book offers a complete toolkit for anyone seeking to improve their health and wellbeing, including meal plans, exercise schedules, and stress-reduction methods.

"Outsmart Fat Fast" is the manual for you if you're sick of the never-ending loop of trendy diets and ineffectual exercise regimens. Join Betty and the numerous others who have improved their lives by realizing the potential of scientifically supported weight reduction.

How is this Book for?

The universe of "**Outsmart Fat Fast: A Definitive Guide to Burning Fat, Boosting Energy, and Balancing Hormones**" is here for you. This book is a thorough guide that will lead you to improved health and well-being, not just another fad diet book.

Why do I need another diet guide? You might be asking yourself as you read this. The reality is that most diet guides emphasize fast fixes and instant weight reduction without considering their long-term impacts on your general health. Our work is unique. To help you lose weight permanently while also enhancing your general health and well-being, we have collected a list of clinically validated techniques and strategies.

Have you ever felt frustrated after attempting various regimens but getting little to no benefit? Or you shed weight and then got it all back, plus some. We know that losing weight can be challenging and stressful, particularly if you lack the necessary knowledge or support. We created this guide for that reason—to arm you with the information and resources you need to defeat fat and reach your health objectives.

Let me tell you a quick tale about Betty, a lady who battled weight issues for a long time. Nothing seemed to work for her, no matter how many diets and weight reduction plans Betty attempted. She was discouraged and believed her weight reduction objectives would never be met. That is until she learned about the techniques and tactics described in this work.

Betty discovered how to better her metabolism, regulate her hormones, and adopt healthy eating practices. She eventually reached her weight loss objectives and began to notice noticeable effects. More significantly, she had never felt happy, healthier, or more energetic.

This book is for anyone who wants to take charge of their health and well-being and is sick of the never-ending pattern of fad diets. Anyone interested in learning how to burn fat, increase vitality, and regulate hormones long-term should read this. This book will give you helpful information and valuable suggestions to help you reach your health objectives, whether you are a novice or a seasoned dieter.

So, this book is for you if you're ready to defeat obesity and take charge of your health and well-being. We have poured our hearts and minds into developing a comprehensive manual that will assist you in reaching your weight reduction objectives and enhancing your general health and well-being.

Let's take this trip together and learn the value of a healthful lifestyle.

This page was left blank intentionally

Introduction: Why Traditional Diets Fail

The fight to reduce weight is a lifelong one for many individuals. They attempt the newest fad diet or weight reduction program every year, only to wind up worse off than they were before. The constraints of conventional diets are the issue, not a lack of discipline or resolve.

Traditional diets frequently call for lowering calories and serving amounts, which can be challenging to maintain over time. People often feel starved, deprived, and irritated due to their frequent use of limitation and deprivation. This method fails to treat the root reasons for weight gain and does not offer a long-term fix.

Furthermore, conventional diets frequently undervalue metabolism and hormone equilibrium's role in weight reduction. Hunger, metabolism, and fat accumulation are all controlled by hormones like insulin, cortisol, and leptin.

Unbalanced levels of these chemicals can cause weight increase and make it challenging to lose weight.

Additionally, conventional diets frequently miss the real reasons for lousy eating behaviors, such as worry, emotional eating, and inadequate sleep. These elements frequently need to be considered in conventional diet plans despite their potential effect on weight and general health.

A novel strategy for shedding pounds and improving general health is required. A holistic strategy that tackles hormone balance, metabolism, and the underlying causes of destructive eating patterns is required rather than a single emphasis on calorie restriction.

We will examine why conventional diets fall short in this book and offer a fresh, science-based strategy for weight reduction and optimum health. We will go in-depth on the significance of hormone balance and metabolism and offer doable plans for reaching and sustaining a healthy weight. We will also discuss the underlying reasons for destructive food patterns and offer practical advice for changing them.

This guide is for anyone ready to change their attitude to their health and wellness and sick of the never-ending cycle of dieting and weight increase. You will have the information and resources necessary to outwit fat quickly and accomplish your health and weight reduction objectives by the conclusion of this book.

This page was left blank intentionally

The science behind fat burning

The human body is a sophisticated mechanism that uses numerous chemical processes to work correctly. Fat combustion is one of the most crucial procedures our body goes through. Fat is kept in our adipose tissue, a form of fibrous tissue. This tissue serves as a storage area for extra energy and is found around and beneath our organs.

When we are in a calorie shortage or physically active, the body utilizes stored fat as fuel. The dissolution of lipids into fatty acids and glycerol is a component of the lipolysis process, which is another name for burning fat. After being carried to the liver, these compounds are transformed into ketone bodies, which the brain and muscles can use as an energy source.

How, though, does the body choose when to retain fat and when to eliminate it? The equilibrium between energy consumption and expenditure is vital to finding the solution. The extra energy is stored as fat when we ingest more calories than we expend. On the other hand, when we expend more calories than we take in, the body is compelled to use fat reserves to make up for the energy shortfall.

Several chemicals greatly influence the regulation of the fat-burning process. The pancreas releases insulin as one of the most crucial hormones in reaction to elevated blood sugar levels. Insulin prevents fat breakdown and encourages storing of glucose as glycogen in the liver and muscles. Low insulin levels increase the likelihood that the body will burn fat as fuel.

Glucagon, a hormone that the pancreas secretes in reaction to reduced blood sugar levels, is another hormone that aids in fat reduction. In addition to promoting the breakdown of fat in fatty tissue, glucose increases the breakdown of glycogen in the liver and muscles. High glucagon levels increase the likelihood that the body will burn fat as fuel.

Adrenaline, cortisol, and growth hormone are additional chemicals that contribute to fat metabolism. In reaction to tension or physical exertion, the adrenal glands release adrenaline, which promotes the breakdown of fat in adipose tissue. The adrenal glands also produce cortisol, which encourages the breakdown of muscular tissue for energy. The pituitary organ secretes growth hormone, which encourages fat decomposition and muscular tissue development.

In addition to hormones, several other variables can affect how fat is burned. These include heredity, maturity, sex, nutrition, and exercise. For instance, while some people have a higher metabolic rate that enables them to expend more calories while at rest, others are naturally prone to store more fat than others. Men typically have more muscle mass and a greater metabolic rate than women, and aging is linked to loss of muscle mass and a slower metabolic rate. Age and sex both affect fat metabolism.

Diet and exercise are crucial components of the fat-burning process. A diet that is high in protein and low in carbs can encourage the burning of fat, whereas a diet that is low in fat and high in carbohydrates can encourage storing fat. By boosting metabolism and releasing chemicals that encourage lipolysis, physical activity, particularly high-intensity exercise, can also aid in fat burning.

This page was left blank intentionally

Common myths about weight loss

A multi-billion-dollar business is dedicated to weight reduction because so many people want an immediate solution to their weight issues. Unfortunately, there are a lot of myths and false beliefs about weight reduction that can cause sadness and despair. This piece will dispel some of the most widespread misconceptions about weight reduction and offer evidence-based recommendations to support your weight loss efforts.

Myth #1: You must eliminate all oil from your diet.

Fat has been vilified for a long time as the adversary of weight reduction. But not all lipids are made equally. Omega-3 fatty acids are crucial for general health and weight reduction, while saturated and trans fats should be avoided. Salmon, avocados, and nuts are just a few meals containing these suitable lipids.

Additionally, eliminating all fat from your diet can make it harder to lose weight. Fat gives people a sense of satiety and aids in blood sugar regulation, which can reduce overeating and sugar desires.

Myth #2: Carbs are bad for you

Like fat, carbohydrates have a bad reputation for contributing to weight increase. But not all carbohydrates are made alike. White bread, sugary beverages, and nibbled foods are highly processed carbohydrates that can cause weight increase and other health issues. However, complex carbohydrates from foods like whole grains, fruits, and veggies are necessary for weight reduction and general wellness.

A full carbohydrate restriction can cause lethargy, headaches, and other unfavorable side effects. For optimum weight reduction, concentrate on ingesting complex carbohydrates in moderation and combining them with protein and healthy fats.

Myth #3: Spot-reducing obesity is possible.

Many think they can target body parts for weight reduction, like their thighs or midsection. This is, unfortunately, not feasible. When you drop weight, your body burns fat throughout, not just in one region.

Focus on overall weight reduction through healthy eating and activity rather than spot-reducing. You will gradually observe that all of your body's fat has decreased.

Myth #4: Following a fad diet is the easiest method to reduce weight.

Fad regimens that promise fast and simple weight reduction to come and go. These diets, however, are frequently unstable and harmful. They may also cause other health issues, such as weight increase.

The best method to reduce weight is through a sustainable, balanced strategy that includes frequent activity and healthy eating. Even though it might take longer, this strategy will result in long-term weight reduction and better general health.

Myth #5: To reduce weight, you must consume fewer calories.

Although a calorie deficit is necessary for weight reduction, this does not inherently entail cutting back on your food intake. Instead, consume more nutrient-dense foods like fruits, veggies, and lean meats. These meals can help you feel filled and satiated while still losing weight because they are high in nutrients and low in calories.

Exercise is another way to boost your calorie expenditure. Your metabolism can be boosted by regular exercise, which will enable you to expend more calories all day long.

Chapter One: The Fat Fast Formula

Hormones in weight loss

They understand how hormones function is crucial for successful and long-lasting weight loss because hormones play a significant part in weight loss. Hormones are chemical signals in the body that control several bodily functions, such as appetite, satiety, and metabolism.

In losing weight, several hormones are involved, including insulin, cortisol, thyroid hormone, leptin, and ghrelin. The pancreas secretes the hormone insulin, which aids in controlling blood sugar levels. Your body creates insulin by consuming carbohydrates to carry glucose into your cells for energy. Weight increase and trouble losing weight are possible consequences of insulin resistance, which happens when the body stops responding to insulin.

The adrenal glands release cortisol, also referred to as the stress hormone, in reaction to worry. Cortisol can boost hunger and desire for fatty, sugary meals, which can result in weight gain. Insulin resistance and a higher chance of type 2 diabetes can result from ongoing stress and elevated cortisol levels.

The thyroid hormone controls metabolism and is essential for weight reduction. Weight gain and trouble losing weight can result from hypothyroidism, a disease in which the thyroid gland does not generate enough thyroid hormone.

Hormones that control appetite and fullness include leptin and ghrelin. Fat cells generate leptin, which tells the brain to eat less and burn more calories. On the other side, the gut produces the hunger-stimulating hormone ghrelin. Overeating and weight increase can result from hormonal imbalances in the body system.

Other hormones, such as testosterone, estrogen, and progesterone, are also involved in weight reduction in addition to these two. The anabolic hormone testosterone helps with fat reduction and muscular gain. The spread of fat is influenced by estrogen and progesterone, which can impact female weight reduction.

Understanding how hormones influence weight loss can create a focused weight-loss strategy that tackles hormonal imbalances. For instance, increasing your fiber and protein intake while decreasing your intake of processed carbs can help improve insulin sensitivity if you have insulin resistance. Yoga and meditation are two stress-reduction practices that can help reduce cortisol levels if you suffer from chronic worry.

In some circumstances, hormone replacement treatment might be required to encourage weight reduction and reestablish hormonal equilibrium. However, it is crucial to consult with a qualified healthcare expert to choose the most appropriate course of action for your particular requirements.

This page was left blank intentionally

Unlocking the Power of Hormones: Your Ultimate Guide to Optimize Fat Burning

Many people only consider food and exercise when reducing weight and burning fat. Hormones play a part in weight reduction, but this is frequently forgotten. Hormones are chemical mediators that control various bodily functions, such as metabolism and fat accumulation. Optimizing your hormones for fat metabolism can make all the difference if you want to lose weight. We will examine the main hormones in fat metabolism in this manual and discuss how to maximize them for the best outcomes.

Hormones and Fat Burning: An Understanding

Hormones are essential for fat metabolism and weight reduction. Insulin, cortisol, growth hormone, and thyroid hormones are the main chemicals in this process. Blood sugar levels are controlled by insulin, which also encourages fat accumulation. The body may struggle to metabolize fat when insulin levels are high because it prefers to store energy. The stress hormone cortisol, particularly in the abdominal region, can also add to fat accumulation. On the other hand, growth hormones and thyroid hormones encourage metabolism and fat loss.

Making Insulin Work Best for Fat Burning

Reducing the intake of refined carbohydrates and sugar is one of the best methods to maximize insulin for fat reduction. These meals raise blood sugar levels, stimulating the release of more insulin and promoting fat accumulation. Instead, concentrate on eating nutrient-dense, whole foods like veggies, lean meats, and healthy fats. Regular exercise, particularly strength training, can also help increase insulin sensitivity and encourage fat reduction.

Cortisol Balance for Fat Burning

Stress management is crucial to maintain a healthy cortisol level and to encourage fat metabolism. Cortisol levels can be lowered by incorporating stress-reduction methods like yoga, meditation, or deep breathing routines. Additionally, getting enough sleep and exercising frequently can help lower tension and encourage fat metabolism.

Increasing Thyroid and Growth Hormones to Promote Fat Burning:

It has been demonstrated that high-intensity interval training (HIIT) encourages growth hormone creation, which may boost fat burning. Additionally, adding weight exercise can help thyroid and growth hormone synthesis. Since protein serves as the building component for muscle tissue, consuming enough protein is also crucial for promoting the creation of these hormones.

Fueling Your Body Right: The Surprising Benefits of a Low-Carb, High-Fat Diet

Low-carb, high-fat diets have become very fashionable in the realm of health and exercise in recent years. These diets, also called ketogenic diets, promote the consumption of healthy fats, modest levels of protein, and little to no carbs.

A low-carb, high-fat diet aims to make ketones, which the liver produces when the body is in ketosis, the body's primary energy source in place of glucose. When the body's glycogen reserves are exhausted, causing it to consume fat for sustenance instead, it enters this metabolic condition.

With this diet, many people have experienced success, noting weight loss, better mental clarity, and greater vitality. In more detail, let's examine the advantages of a low-carb, high-fat diet.

Weight loss: It has been demonstrated that a low-carb, high-fat diet can help people lose weight, particularly those who are overweight or obese. The body is more effective at consuming fat for energy when it is in a condition of ketosis, which may result in a decrease in body fat. Additionally, high-fat foods are typically more filling than high-carb foods, which can result in a decrease in daily calorie consumption. More significant weight reduction and better body composition may come from this.

Improved blood sugar regulation: Glucose, produced when carbohydrates are broken down, is used by the body as energy. However, eating an excessive amount of carbs can result in high blood sugar levels, which can be harmful to health.

By lowering the quantity of glucose in the bloodstream, a low-carb, high-fat diet can assist people with blood sugar control. People with diabetes or metabolic syndrome may benefit from this in particular.

Increased energy: Many individuals who adopt a low-carb, high-fat diet say they have more energy. This is due to the increased body capacity to utilize fat for energy, which can offer a steady energy supply throughout the day. Additionally, high-fat foods typically contain more nutrients per serving than high-carbohydrate foods, boosting energy levels and enhancing general health.

Enhanced mental clarity: Some people claim that eating a diet high in fat and low in carbohydrates helps them think more clearly. This might be because ketones can give the brain a more consistent energy supply, enhancing cognitive performance.

A high-fat diet can also aid in reducing inflammation in the brain, which has been connected to diseases like Alzheimer's and melancholy.

Reduced inflammation: A low-carb, high-fat diet has been demonstrated to reduce inflammation in the body, a component in many chronic illnesses.
Inflammation is the body's normal reaction to damage or illness, but persistent inflammation can result in the onset of diseases like cancer, heart disease, and arthritis.

A low-carb, high-fat diet can aid in decreasing inflammation and enhancing general health by reducing carbohydrate ingestion and increasing the consumption of beneficial fats.

In summation, there are numerous advantages to a low-carb, high-fat diet for general health and well-being. This kind of diet can assist people in achieving their health and exercise objectives by encouraging weight reduction and decreasing inflammation.

Before beginning a low-carb, high-fat diet, as with any diet, it is essential to speak with a healthcare professional, particularly if you have any underlying medical issues. However, for many people, this kind of food can be a potent instrument for adequately nourishing the body and bringing out its maximum potential.

This page was left blank intentionally

Chapter Two: Eat the Right Fats

Healthy vs unhealthy fats

Fat is a crucial substance that gives the body energy, aids in vitamin absorption, and is essential for keeping good skin and hair. But not all fats are made alike; if eaten in excess, some fats can be bad for our health. The distinctions between good and unhealthy fats and how they impact our general health will be covered in this piece.

What are good fats?

Unsaturated fats in fatty seafood and plant-based foods are considered healthy lipids. They have a variety of health advantages, including lowering inflammation, enhancing heart health, and fostering brain function. They are necessary for the body to operate correctly. Monounsaturated and polyunsaturated lipids are the two major categories of healthy fats.

Individualized Fats

When cooled, monounsaturated lipids solidify after being liquid at ambient temperature. Foods like almonds, seeds, avocados, and veggie oils contain them. According to research, monounsaturated fats can help lower levels of poor cholesterol (LDL) and raise good cholesterol (HDL) levels, decreasing the chance of heart disease. They also aid in reducing the chance of type 2 diabetes and blood pressure.

Unsaturated Fats, Poly

Nuts, seeds, and veggie oils are examples of plant-based meals that contain polyunsaturated fats, which are also liquid at room temperature. They are further divided into omega-3 and omega-6 fatty acid categories.

It has been demonstrated that omega-3 fatty acids in fatty fish like salmon and tuna decrease inflammation, enhance cognitive performance, and lower the chance of heart disease. The body needs omega-6 fatty acids to operate correctly, but they should only be taken in amounts and can be found in foods like nuts and vegetable oils.

Why are some fats unhealthy?

Saturated and trans fats, which are typically found in processed foods and goods derived from animals, are unhealthy lipids. If eaten in excess, these lipids can raise harmful cholesterol levels and cause various health issues.

Unhealthy Fats

Saturated lipids are typically found in animal-based goods like beef and dairy and are solid at ambient temperature. They have been connected to higher amounts of bad cholesterol (LDL) and a higher chance of diabetes, heart disease, and stroke.

No Trans Fats

Hydrogen is chemically added to liquid veggie oils to produce trans fats, which are more solid and convenient for cooking. They are frequently discovered in prepared foods like margarine, cooked foods, and baked products. Trans lipids have been found to raise levels of bad cholesterol

(LDL) and lower levels of good cholesterol (HDL), which increases the chance of heart disease.

Comparing excellent and unhealthy fats

The chemical makeup of healthy and harmful lipids is what distinguishes them most. Unsaturated bonds, which are more fluid in healthy lipids, let the fat stay liquid at room temperature. Conversely, unhealthy fats have stiffer, more inflexible saturated bonds that harden at ambient temperature.

Consuming healthy fats in balance has several health advantages for the body, including lowering inflammation, enhancing cardiac health, and enhancing cognitive function. Conversely, eating too many unhealthy lipids can increase weight, heart disease and other health issues.

Fuel Up for Fat Burn: Your Guide to Foods That Aid or Hinder Optimal Weight Loss

Your diet can either be a friend or an adversary when losing weight. You can attain your ideal body weight by consuming foods that encourage optimal fat burning, but eating the wrong foods can make weight reduction much more challenging. This article will examine the meals that can support or undermine your efforts to lose weight.

What to Eat to Burn Fat Optimally

Lean Proteins: Consuming lean proteins like poultry, fish, turkey, and tofu can aid in weight loss and muscular growth. Additionally, protein is nourishing, which can make you feel fuller for longer and help you consume fewer calories altogether.

Fruits and veggies are abundant in fiber, vitamins, and nutrients that can support your efforts to lose weight. They also have antioxidants, which lessen inflammation, a factor in weight increase.

Whole Grains: Whole grains have a high fiber content and can help control blood sugar levels. Examples of whole grains include brown rice, quinoa, and whole wheat bread. This lessens the chance of insulin surges, which can lead to fat accumulation.

Nuts and seeds: Nuts and seeds contain fiber, protein, and suitable lipids. They can help you stay satiated and filled while giving your body the necessary nutrients.

Healthy Fats: Healthy fats, like oily seafood, avocados, and olive oil, can help lower inflammation and encourage fat metabolism. They also aid in preserving your sense of satiety and fullness.

Foods to Stay Away from for Best Fat Burning

Foods that have been processed include crisps, biscuits, and sweets, which are frequently high in sugar, bad fats, and calories. These meals can contribute to weight increase and other health issues.

Sugary beverages: Sugary beverages have a lot of calories and sugar, pop, and juice. Both insulin intolerance and weight increase may result from them.

White Flour and Refined Carbs: Consuming white flour and refined carbohydrates, such as those found in white noodles, bread, and pastries, can cause insulin to rise and lead to weight gain.

Fried Foods: Fried foods frequently contain high calories and harmful lipids, which can lead to weight increase and other health issues.

High-Fat Dairy Goods: Dairy goods with high-fat content, like cheese and butter, can be very calorie- and fat-rich. Excessive consumption of these items can cause weight increase and other health issues.

Conclusion

The foods you consume can have a significant impact on weight reduction. You can attain your ideal body weight and enhance your general health by eating foods that help you eliminate fat. On the other hand, eating meals that prevent fat metabolism can make it much harder to lose weight. By making wise dietary decisions, you can adequately fuel your body and achieve the best weight reduction outcomes.

This page was left blank intentionally

Fat Fuel: Unleashing the Power of MCT Oil and Other Healthy Fats for Optimal Health

People have long believed that lipids are unhealthy for the body and should be shunned. Recent research has revealed that some fats are good for our health, and not all are detrimental. One of these healthy lipids that have been getting recognition because of its possible health advantages is a medium-chain triglyceride (MCT) oil. In this piece, we will examine the advantages of MCT oil and other healthy fat sources and how they can promote our health at their best.

The Advantages of MCT Oil: MCT oil is a form of heavy fat in dairy products, coconut oil, and palm oil. In contrast to other kinds of fat, MCT oil is quickly broken down by the body and turned into ketones, which the body and brain can use as an alternative energy source. The following are some possible advantages of MCT oil:

Weight reduction: According to studies, MCT oil can reduce weight by raising satiety levels, lowering calorie consumption, and accelerating metabolism.

MCT oil has been proven to enhance brain performance in individuals with Alzheimer's disease and mild cognitive impairment.

Improved Exercise Performance: MCT oil has been demonstrated to improve exercise performance by giving the muscles a fast energy supply.

Reduced Inflammation: MCT oil has anti-inflammatory qualities that may help lessen the body's inflammation, a risk factor for several chronic illnesses.

Other Healthy Fat Sources: For the best possible health, we should include other healthy fat sources in our food besides MCT oil. Here are a few instances:

Avocado: Avocado is an excellent source of monounsaturated fats, which have been associated with better heart health and reduced amounts of LDL cholesterol (also known as "bad" cholesterol").

Nuts and Seeds: Nuts and seeds are full of fiber, protein, and polyunsaturated and monounsaturated fats, which can aid in weight reduction and enhance cardiac health.

Fatty Fish: Omega-3 fatty acids, abundant in fatty fish like salmon, mackerel, and sardines, have been associated with improved heart health, decreased inflammation, and enhanced cognitive performance.

Conclusion: There are many health advantages to including healthy lipids in our diet, such as MCT oil, avocado, nuts and seeds, and oily seafood. Healthy fats can help us reach our objectives, whether they involve weight loss, enhancing brain function, increasing workout efficiency, or lowering inflammation.

So, let's remember to include some healthy fats the next time we prepare our meals to fuel our bodies and encourage optimum health properly.

This page was left blank intentionally

Chapter Three: Ditch the Carbs

Carbs and Fat: The Insulin Connection

There has long been controversy surrounding carbs and fat in nutrition and wellness. Others abide by low-carb diets for the same reason, but many think cutting back on fat is the secret to losing weight. However, the connection between carbohydrates and fat is a lot more nuanced than it might first appear.

Insulin, an essential hormone in controlling blood sugar levels, is one of the most significant variables in this relationship. Upon ingestion, carbs are converted to glucose and discharged into the bloodstream. Blood sugar levels rise as a result, which causes the pancreas to produce insulin. Glucose can be used for energy in our cells by being transported from circulation by insulin.

Insulin aids in regulating the body's fat accumulation, which is one of its additional crucial roles. High insulin levels increase the body's propensity to retain extra energy as fat. This is due to insulin telling the body to use carbohydrates instead of fat as its primary energy source. Therefore, you may be more likely to lose weight and retain fat if you consume a high-carb diet that frequently increases your insulin levels.

On the other hand, consuming fewer carbohydrates can significantly affect hormone levels and fat accumulation. Your body generates less insulin when you follow a low-carb diet, making it less likely to retain extra calories as fat. Because of this, many individuals discover that they can drop weight more quickly on a low-carb diet than on a high-carb diet.

Not all carbohydrates have the same effects on insulin levels, so keeping that in mind is essential. Simple carbohydrates, like those in sweet foods and beverages, tend to cause blood sugar and insulin levels to rise more quickly than complex carbohydrates, like those in whole cereals and veggies. As a result, it's crucial to concentrate on reducing your consumption of essential carbs rather than complicated ones if you want to lower your carb intake to help control insulin and fat accumulation.

This page was left blank intentionally

Cutting Carbs: Tips for Safe and Effective Reduction

The body's primary source of energy is carbohydrates or carbs. However, eating too many carbohydrates can increase weight and cause other health problems. Individuals frequently use low-carb diets to reduce their carb consumption and achieve weight reduction objectives. But carbohydrate consumption must be safely reduced to keep a nutritious and well-balanced diet.

We'll look at advice for safety and successfully reducing carbs in this piece.

Before beginning a carbohydrate diet reduction, establish attainable and realistic objectives for you. Expecting to eliminate all carbohydrates immediately is unrealistic and untenable. Reduce carb consumption gradually by 10% each week until you achieve your goal.

Concentrate on high-quality carbohydrates: Not all carbohydrates are made alike. Certain carbohydrates, such as those in fruits, veggies, and whole grains, are nutritious and healthful energy sources. Others, like those in processed meals and sugary beverages, are harmful and cause weight increases. Limit your consumption of low-quality carbohydrates and put your attention on high-quality carbs.

Include protein and good fats: When cutting back on your consumption of carbohydrates, it's essential to swap out those calories for other nutrients like protein and good fats. This will make you feel content and satiated, lessening your desire for carbohydrate-rich foods. Lean meats, seafood, eggs, and plant-based proteins like beans and tofu are all excellent forms of protein. Foods like bananas, nuts, and olive oil contain healthy lipids.

Plan your meals: A meal schedule can help you stay on track with your low-carb objectives. Look for dishes rich in protein and good fats and limited in carbohydrates. Make an inventory of the items you'll need for your dinners and go buying with it. You can also save time and money by doing this.

Don't overlook fiber: Fiber is a crucial nutrient that supports healthy digestion and can make you feel satiated and filled. Ensure you're still consuming enough fiber from foods like veggies, fruits, and whole cereals when you reduce your carb consumption.

Keep hydrated: Drinking plenty of water can aid digestion and help you feel satiated and filled. Aim to consume at least 8 glasses of water daily and avoid pop and fruit juice.

Pay attention to carb substitutes: Using manufactured low-carb foods and artificial sweets is common when cutting back on carbohydrates. However, these goods might be harmful and lead to weight increase. Instead, emphasize whole meals and moderate use of natural sugars like honey and maple syrup.

In summary, cutting back on carbohydrates can help you lose weight and generally get healthier. You can safely and successfully decrease your carb consumption and reach your health goals by establishing reasonable objectives, concentrating on high-quality carbohydrates, integrating protein and healthy fats, organizing your meals, consuming enough fiber, staying hydrated, and being aware of carb alternatives.

Intermittent fasting

A common nutritional strategy called intermittent fasting (IF) includes alternating fasting and eating times. It has been around for millennia and performed for diverse purposes by different cultures and religions. It has recently grown in favor due to its possible health advantages, which include longevity, better blood sugar management, and weight loss.

The 16/8 technique, the 5:2 diet, and alternate-day fasting are the three most popular forms of intermittent fasting, though there are others. The 16/8 technique calls for a daily 8-hour eating interval after 16 hours of fasting. In the 5:2 diet, participants regularly consume for five days while limiting their daily caloric consumption to 500–600 calories for the remaining two. Every other day, participants in the alternate-day fast observe a 24-hour fast.

The biochemical condition known as ketosis is what intermittent fasting causes to occur. When the body runs out of glucose for fuel, it enters a state of ketosis and begins converting stored fat into ketones for use as fuel.

This condition is comparable to that brought on by a high-fat, low-carb diet.

Weight reduction is one of the advantages of irregular fasting. People can produce a calorie imbalance by consuming fewer calories overall, which may result in weight reduction. Additionally, the body may expend more calories at rest due to irregular fasting because it has a higher metabolic rate. Studies have shown intermittent fasting can be as effective for weight reduction and changing body shape as constant calorie limitation.

Additionally, intermittent fasting may enhance blood sugar regulation. According to studies, it can increase insulin sensitivity in cells, lower blood sugar levels, and lessen insulin resistance. For those at risk of getting type 2 diabetes or those who already have it, this can be especially helpful.

Additionally, there may be anti-aging benefits to irregular fasting. It has been demonstrated through studies on animals that it can lengthen life and postpone the start of age-related illnesses. The cell processes that support cellular healing and regeneration may have been activated.

For the majority of individuals, intermittent fasting is usually safe. It is crucial to remember that it might not be appropriate for everyone, especially for people with specific medical conditions, pregnant or nursing women, and kids. A healthcare professional should always be consulted before beginning any nutritional strategy.

Chapter Four: Get Moving

Getting Fit Matters

Did you know that regular exercise can aid in fat burning? Regular exercise is frequently advised as a crucial element of a healthy lifestyle. Exercise can boost calorie expenditure and aid in weight loss with a healthy diet and lifestyle. In this piece, we'll talk about the advantages of fitness for burning fat.

Higher Calorie Burn

The number of calories expended by the body rises with exercise. When you exercise, your body needs the energy to power the action. These accumulated body fat calories provide this energy. Your body consumes more calories when you work out more vigorously. This rise in calorie expenditure can aid in generating the calorie deficit required for fat reduction.

Better Metabolism

The method by which your body transforms food into energy, known as metabolism, is improved by exercise. Your body will be better able to consume calories and fat even at leisure if your metabolism is quicker. Resistance exercise can also aid in gaining lean muscle mass, boosting metabolism and fat reduction even more.

Diminished inflammation

Although inflammation is a normal reaction to injury or sickness, it can persist over time and cause various health issues, including weight increase and trouble losing weight. Exercise has been demonstrated to lower inflammatory levels in the body, enhancing fat metabolism and improving general health.

Increased Sensitivity to Insulin

A hormone called insulin controls the body's blood sugar levels. Insulin resistance, which develops when the body's sensitivity to insulin decreases, can cause weight increase and make it challenging to lose weight. Exercise has been demonstrated to increase insulin sensitivity, which may aid in the body's improved control of blood sugar levels and fat burning.

Stress management

Stress can negatively affect both physical and emotional health. It can also cause weight increase and make it more challenging to lose weight. Exercise has been shown to boost happiness and lower tension levels, supporting fat burning and encouraging a healthy lifestyle.

Exercise that promotes fat loss

Any healthy lifestyle must include exercise because it is crucial to encouraging fat metabolism and weight loss. Regular exercise can help raise metabolic rate, burn more calories, and decrease body fat when paired with a healthy diet. To promote fat reduction, however, not all exercises are similarly beneficial. This piece will discuss some of the top exercises for losing weight and how to work them into your daily exercise regimen.

Training with High-Intensity Intervals (HIIT)

High-intensity bursts of action alternate with relaxation intervals in HIIT, a type of cardiovascular exercise. As it helps raise metabolic rate and expend calories during and after the activity, this exercise is especially effective at encouraging fat reduction.

One research showed that HIIT was more efficient than conventional steady-state cardio at reducing body fat. It was published in the International Journal of Obesity. Compared to those who did steady-state exercise, HIIT participants dropped more fat and improved their cardiovascular endurance more.

Resistance Exercise

Another efficient strategy to encourage fat reduction is resistance training, weightlifting, or strength training. Resistance exercise includes using weights or resistance bands to improve strength and muscular density. You'll expend more calories even when you're not moving because adding muscle increases your resting metabolic rate.

Resistance training was found to be efficient at decreasing body fat and boosting lean body mass in both men and women, according to research released in the Journal of Applied Physiology. Resistance training was found to be more efficient at decreasing abdominal obesity than aerobic exercise in different research that was released in the journal Obesity.

Walking

Even though walking may not seem incredibly challenging, it can still help you lose weight. One research found that strolling for 30 minutes a day, five days a week, for 12 weeks significantly reduced body fat in overweight and obese women. The study was published in the Journal of Exercise Nutrition and Biochemistry.

Low-impact exercise like walking is simple to fit into your everyday schedule. You can take the steps rather than lifting, strolling to work, or walking briskly during your lunch break.

Cycling is yet another powerful strategy to encourage weight reduction. Cycling can help boost metabolism, expend calories, and decrease body weight, whether you prefer to ride outside or on a stationary bike.

One research showed that cycling helped overweight and obese women improve their cardiovascular fitness and reduce their body fat. The study was released in the Journal of Sports Science and Medicine.

Interval Training

With little to no rest in between, several movements are performed back-to-back during circuit training. Due to its ability to boost metabolism and expend calories, this exercise can be especially effective at encouraging fat reduction.

According to one research in the Journal of Strength and Conditioning Research, people who are overweight or obese can benefit from circuit training by losing body fat and gaining lean body mass.

Including fat-burning activities in your fitness regimen can assist you in losing weight and enhancing your general health. Always check with your doctor before beginning a new fitness regimen, particularly if you have any medical issues.

This page was left blank intentionally

Breaking Through Barriers: Overcoming Obstacles to Exercise

It cannot be easy to fit fitness into your everyday schedule. There are many causes for why individuals frequently fail to maintain a fitness routine. These obstacles can make starting or maintaining consistency challenging, whether it be a shortage of time, desire, or resources. It's crucial to understand that these challenges are surmountable. In this piece, we'll talk about some typical fitness obstacles and offer advice on how to get past them.

Limited time

Lack of time is one of the biggest obstacles to exercise. Finding time to exercise can seem impossible with a job, family duties, and other commitments. But even brief fitness sessions can have a significant effect on your health. Think about scheduling your exercise sessions throughout the day in smaller, more doable chunks. For instance, consider going for a 10-minute stroll during your lunch break or fitting in a 20-minute workout right before work.

Not Being Motivated

Another typical obstacle to exercise is a need for more desire. Finding the motivation to work out frequently can be difficult, particularly if you do not immediately see any effects. But desire can be developed. Try establishing and monitoring attainable objectives for yourself. To add social support and accountability to your routine, consider finding an exercise buddy or enrolling in a fitness program.

The absence of resources

A lack of resources, such as a club subscription or exercise gear, can significantly hamper exercise. But many methods exist to work out without spending much money or needing a gym subscription. Squats and push-ups can be performed anywhere, and many internet fitness videos and applications can be used with little to no equipment.

Anxiety of Injury

Another frequent obstacle to exercise is the fear of getting hurt, especially for those new to it or with a history of accidents. But beginning with low-impact workouts and progressively stepping up the intensity and challenge can help avoid injury. Working with a physical therapist or personal trainer can also offer direction on correct form and technique, even lowering the risk of harm.

Not enough energy

Finding the motivation to exercise can be difficult if you're exhausted. Exercise, on the other hand, can genuinely boost vitality and lessen fatigue. Try beginning with low-intensity exercises, like yoga or a stroll, and progressively raising intensity as your energy levels increase if lack of energy is a significant obstacle.

Weather circumstances

The last major obstacle to exercise is the weather, especially for people who prefer outdoor sports. But regardless of the weather, there are plenty of interior fitness choices, including at-home exercises and club programs.

This page was left blank intentionally

Chapter Five: Fat and Metabolism

Why You Need Fat in the Body

The first thing that typically comes to mind when most people think of fat is frequently something terrible, such as weight increase, unhealthy eating patterns, and an unattractive body form. But it's crucial to remember that not all fats are identical. Fat is a necessary substance for preserving general health and well-being. In this piece, we'll discuss the various kinds of fat and why your body needs them.

What is Fat?

Let's describe fat first before exploring why it is crucial. Along with proteins and carbs, fat is a component that gives the body energy. It is made up of compounds called fatty acids, which are comprised of carbon, hydrogen, and oxygen atoms. Saturated, unsaturated, and trans fats are the three significant kinds of fatty acids that can be identified.

Why Your Body Needs Fat

Delivers Energy

The body's primary source of energy is fat. When you eat, your body converts the dietary lipids into fatty acids, which are then brought to the liver, turning them into energy. The body then uses this energy for various purposes, such as movement, temperature regulating, and assisting organ function.

Ensures Brain Health

Since the brain is about 60% fat, it requires a steady amount of fat to operate correctly. The shape and operation of brain cells are crucially maintained by the fatty acids in fat. Fat also contributes to the formation of the myelin layer, which protects nerve cells and facilitates effective neuronal transmission.

Taking in vitamins

The fat-soluble vitamins A, D, E, and K must break down into fat for the body to receive them. These micronutrients wouldn't be taken and used by the body if fat didn't exist.

These vitamins are essential for preserving strong bones, epidermis, vision, and immune systems.

vital organs

Additionally, fat acts as a cushion to safeguard the body's tissues. It protects delicate systems like the heart, liver, and kidneys to prevent harm and injury.

controls hormones

Chemical mediators called hormones are in charge of controlling several physiological processes. A form of fat called cholesterol creates several hormones, including estradiol and testosterone. The body cannot correctly make and control these hormones without fat.

Variety of Fat

Some kinds of fat are better than others; not all fats are made alike. There are three significant categories of fat:

Unhealthy Fat

Animal goods like meat, cheese, and eggs typically contain saturated fat. It can also be discovered in some plant-based forms like coconut and palm oil since it is solid at room temperature and raises the risk of heart disease and other health issues when overeating; saturated fat is frequently called "bad" fat.

Reduced Saturation

Olive oil, almonds, seeds, olives, and other plant-based foods are familiar sources of unsaturated fat. It is liquid at ambient temperature, and because it can help lower cholesterol levels and the chance of heart disease, it is frequently referred to as "good" fat.

Added Fat

Trans fat is a form of fat produced when partly hydrogenating liquid vegetable oils, which causes the oils to solidify at room temperature. Processed foods like baked products, fried foods, and nibbled foods are frequently high in trans-fat. Because it can elevate cholesterol levels and increase the chance of heart disease, it is considered the worst fat form.

This page was left blank intentionally

Misconception about metabolism

The word metabolism concerns energy levels, weight reduction, and general wellness. It's no secret that quicker metabolism is frequently considered a positive quality because it's thought to produce more energy, boost fat burning, and result in a more petite frame. However, numerous myths about metabolism can be deceiving and impede people from reaching their exercise and health objectives. In this piece, we'll look at some of the most widespread myths about metabolism and what the science honestly states.

Myth #1: Metabolism is a permanent characteristic

One of the biggest myths about metabolism is that it's a set characteristic that can't be altered. Although some individuals can have a quicker or slower metabolism than others inherently, many other variables can affect metabolisms, such as nutrition, exercise, sleep quality, and stress levels.

Resistance exercise, for instance, has been shown to increase muscle density and speed up metabolism even when the subject is at rest. The thermic effect, or the energy needed to process and assimilate nutrients from food, is another way that eating a diet rich in protein and fiber can speed up metabolism.

Myth #2: Consuming short, regular meals speeds up metabolism

Unlike another prevalent misconception about metabolism, eating little and often can increase metabolism and aid in weight reduction. Regular meals can help control blood sugar levels and avoid overeating, but there isn't much proof to support the claim that it also speeds up metabolism.

Studies have revealed that the regularity of meals has little impact on metabolism and weight reduction. The total amount of calories eaten and the caloric quality is more significant.

Myth #3: Supplements for weight loss increase metabolism

Many weight reduction supplements promise to increase metabolism and promote fat burning, but most of these claims lack empirical backing. Even though some ingredients, like caffeine and green tea extract, may slightly impact metabolism, the effect is typically transient. It may not be strong enough to support long-term weight reduction.

Furthermore, the FDA does not control many weight reduction supplements, which may contain harmful components detrimental to health.

Myth #4: Fasting causes the metabolism to slow down.

Fasting, or depriving oneself of food for an extended period, is frequently perceived as a bad habit that can slow down metabolism and cause muscle loss. However, studies have shown that fasting briefly can increase metabolism and encourage fat reduction.

Particularly intermittent fasting has been shown to boost metabolism and encourage weight reduction while offering additional health advantages like better blood sugar regulation and decreased inflammation.

Myth #5: The metabolism slows down in the starvation state

Many think severely cutting calories can result in "starvation mode," where the body slows down the metabolism to preserve energy. While it is true that calorie restriction can cause the metabolism to slow down, this impact is typically only noticed in severe, prolonged instances of calorie restriction.

In most instances, a moderate calorie reduction can result in weight loss and better health. It is also rare to substantially slow down metabolism.

Metabolism: The Key to Effective Weight Loss

Metabolic rate is undoubtedly a topic you've heard about if you attempt to lose weight. Many people think metabolism is the secret to losing weight, but what is metabolism, and how does it impact weight loss?

Your body uses the metabolic process to turn sustenance into energy. It's a multifaceted process that includes numerous biochemical reactions and is affected by various variables, including your age, sex, weight, and level of exercise.

Your diet's composition has an impact on your metabolism as well. Protein and fiber are two foods that can speed up your metabolism and help you expend more calories, while processed foods and sugary beverages can cause your metabolism to slow down and cause you to gain weight.

How does metabolism impact calorie burning?

Since your metabolism controls how many calories your body consumes each day, it is essential for weight reduction. You will acquire weight if you ingest more calories than your body can expend, and you will drop weight if you do the opposite.

The basal metabolic rate is one mechanism by which metabolism influences weight reduction. (BMR). Your body uses calories at rest to sustain essential physiological processes like respiration and blood circulation, and this figure is known as your BMR.

Several variables, such as age, sex, weight, and body makeup, impact your basal metabolic rate (BMR). Your BMR typically decreases with advancing age, which may make weight loss more challenging. People with more muscle mass tend to have a greater BMR than those with less muscle mass, and women typically have a slower BMR than males.

It would help if you consumed fewer calories than your body burns to generate a calorie deficit and drop weight. You can achieve this by consuming fewer calories, becoming more active, or doing both simultaneously.

However, if you drastically cut calories, your body may lower your metabolism to save energy. This may make it more challenging to reduce weight and, in some instances, may even result in weight gain.

It's critical to keep a modest calorie deficit, a healthy diet, and an exercise program to prevent this. Without putting your body into "starvation mode," this can help increase metabolism and encourage weight reduction.

Can you increase your metabolism to burn more calories?

There is no secret trick to increase your metabolism; contrary to popular belief, you cannot increase your metabolism to reduce weight. You can, however, take a few steps to support a healthy metabolism and encourage weight reduction.

Increasing muscle mass is one of the most excellent methods to speed up your metabolism. Since muscle consumes more calories than fat throughout the day, including at rest, the more muscle you have, the more calories you expend.

A meal rich in protein and carbohydrates can also help you speed up your metabolism. Because protein has a solid thermic impact, your body uses more calories to process it than it does to break down fat or carbohydrates. By encouraging satiety and lowering your total calorie consumption, fiber can also help speed up your metabolism.

Finally, frequent exercise can help increase your metabolism by building muscle and encouraging fat-burning. High-intensity interval training (HIIT) has successfully increased metabolism and fostered weight loss.

Chapter Six: Underlying Issues

Hidden Health Issues Hindering Weight Loss

Many individuals find it challenging to lose weight; occasionally, underlying medical conditions can make it even harder. Consider whether an underlying health issue may be causing your weight loss difficulties if you've been battling to lose weight despite eating a healthy diet and exercising frequently.

Hormonal abnormalities, sleep difficulties, and digestive problems are just a few of the medical conditions that can make it more challenging to drop weight. We'll look at a few of these ailments and how they may impact weight reduction in this piece.

Abnormalities in hormones

Hormones heavily influence weight control, and imbalances in some hormones can make it more challenging to reduce weight. Insulin, a hormone that controls blood sugar levels and aids in hunger regulation, is especially crucial for weight reduction.

A common hormonal imbalance known as insulin resistance, which happens when the body becomes less receptive to insulin, can cause a weight increase and make it more challenging to reduce weight. It can also be difficult to lose weight if there are other hormonal abnormalities, like poor thyroid function or elevated cortisol levels.

It's crucial to consult your healthcare practitioner if you believe a hormonal disorder may cause difficulty in losing weight. They can request blood tests to determine your hormone levels and, if required, suggest the proper course of action.

Problems of sleep

- Sleep is essential for maintaining good health and is crucial for controlling weight. According to studies, those who don't get enough sleep are more likely to be overweight or fat and may find it more challenging to lose weight.

- Lack of sleep can interfere with chemicals that control food and metabolism, increasing hunger and lowering energy consumption, which is one explanation for this. Fatigue brought on by lack of sleep can make it challenging to maintain a healthy diet and exercise regimen.

- It's crucial to consult your healthcare practitioner if you have difficulty losing weight and exhibiting signs of a sleep problem, such as snoring, insomnia, or excessive daily sleepiness. They suggest a sleep analysis to identify a sleep problem and suggest the best action.

Digestive problems

Because they can interfere with the usage of nutrients from food, digestive problems can also make it more challenging to drop weight. Irritable bowel syndrome (IBS), celiac disease, and inflammatory bowel disease (IBD) are a few conditions that can interfere with nutritional intake and digestion.

Nutrient deficiencies and weight loss may result from the autoimmune disorder celiac disease, which impairs the body's capacity to process gluten. Malabsorption and weight loss may also result from IBD, which encompasses diseases like Crohn's disease and ulcerative colitis.

By making it more challenging to maintain a healthy diet and exercise schedule, IBS, a prevalent digestive condition marked by stomach discomfort, bloating, and changes in bowel patterns, can hinder weight reduction. People with IBS may need to avoid specific meals that worsen their symptoms to get all the nutrients they require for weight reduction.

It's crucial to consult your healthcare practitioner if you think a stomach problem may be causing your difficulty in losing weight. They can request tests to identify the underlying problem and suggest the best course of action.

Winning the Battle Against Hypothyroidism and Insulin Resistance

Insulin intolerance and hypothyroidism are medical disorders that can significantly affect your general health and well-being. Both conditions can increase weight and make it more challenging to reduce weight, but you can control and treat them properly.

The proper method to deal with hypothyroidism and insulin resistance will be discussed in this piece, along with lifestyle modifications and available therapies.

Hypothyroidism

The thyroid gland's inability to make enough thyroid hormone, which is necessary for controlling metabolism, results in hypothyroidism. Weight gain, fatigue, and other signs result from the body's metabolism slowing down when thyroid hormone levels are insufficient.

It's crucial to emphasize healthy food and a way of living to fight hypothyroidism. One way to achieve this is to consume a healthy diet high in fruits, veggies, whole grains, and lean protein. Additionally, it's crucial to stay away from processed foods, sweetened beverages, and excessive alcohol consumption, all of which can exacerbate the signs of hypothyroidism and promote inflammation.

Exercise regularly is also crucial for controlling hyperthyroidism. Exercise can help increase energy levels, speed up metabolism, and reduce weight. On most days of the week, try to get at least 30 minutes of moderate-intensity exercises, such as brisk strolling, riding, or swimming.

Medication may also be required to address hypothyroidism and dietary and behavioral modifications. Hypothyroidism is a prevalent condition that can be treated with thyroid hormone replacement therapy, which includes taking synthetic thyroid hormones to make up for what the body isn't making. To guarantee the best possible care, your doctor can decide on the correct dose and track your thyroid hormone levels over time.

Insulin sensitivity

The situation known as insulin resistance occurs when the body becomes less receptive to the hormone insulin, which is crucial for controlling blood sugar levels. The body's cells are less able to take glucose from the bloodstream when insulin resistance develops, which raises blood sugar levels and causes weight increases.

It's crucial to emphasize healthy food and lifestyle to fight insulin resistance. One way to achieve this is to consume a healthy diet high in fiber-rich foods like fruits, veggies, whole grains, and legumes. Additionally, it's critical to stay away from processed and sugary meals, which can exacerbate insulin resistance and cause blood sugar surges.

The management of insulin intolerance also requires regular exercise. Exercise can help encourage weight reduction and increase insulin sensitivity. On most days of the week, try to get at least 30 minutes of moderate-intensity exercises, such as brisk strolling, riding, or swimming.

Medication may also be required to address insulin resistance and dietary and behavioral modifications. Metformin is a popular drug for treating insulin resistance, which lessens glucose production in the liver and increases insulin sensitivity. Your doctor can determine the correct dose and continuously check your blood sugar levels to guarantee the best possible care.

Unlocking Optimal Health: The Benefits of Working with a Pro

Taking care of your health is one of the most important things you can do for yourself. It's no secret that a healthy diet, regular exercise, and good sleep habits are all essential for achieving optimal health. But did you know that working with a healthcare professional can take your health to the next level? This article will explore the benefits of working with a healthcare professional and how they can help you achieve optimal health.

What is a healthcare professional?

A healthcare professional is a licensed individual who has received specialized training in a specific area of healthcare. Examples of healthcare professionals include doctors, nurses, dietitians, physical therapists, and psychologists, among others. These professionals have the knowledge and expertise to help individuals improve their health and well-being through various means, including medical treatment, counseling, and lifestyle modifications.

Benefits of working with a healthcare professional

Personalized care

One of the primary benefits of working with healthcare professionals is that they provide personalized care. This means they take the time to get to know you, your medical history, and your health goals. They can then develop a personalized treatment plan tailored to your needs and circumstances.

Expert knowledge

Healthcare professionals have extensive knowledge and expertise in their respective areas of healthcare. They can provide accurate information and advice on various health-related topics, including disease prevention, healthy lifestyle habits, and medical treatments. This knowledge can be invaluable in helping you make informed decisions about your health.

Monitoring and follow-up

Another benefit of working with a healthcare professional is that they can monitor your progress and provide follow-up care. This is especially important for individuals with chronic conditions, as ongoing monitoring can help ensure the condition is managed correctly and complications are avoided.

Improved outcomes

Working with a healthcare professional can also lead to improved health outcomes. Studies have shown that individuals who work with healthcare professionals have better health outcomes than those who do not. Healthcare professionals can provide the expertise, guidance, and support needed for optimal health.

Accountability

Finally, working with a healthcare professional can provide a sense of accountability. When you have someone to report to and who is invested in your health, you may be more motivated to stick to healthy habits and make positive changes.

Types of Healthcare professionals

There are many types of healthcare professionals, each with its area of expertise. Here are a few examples:

Doctors: Doctor are licensed healthcare professionals specializing in diagnosing and treating medical conditions. They can provide various medical treatments, including medications, procedures, and surgeries.

Nurses: Nurses are licensed healthcare professionals who provide various healthcare services, including administering medications, monitoring vital signs, and providing patient education.

Dietitians: Dietitians are healthcare professionals who specialize in nutrition. They can provide personalized nutrition plans to help individuals achieve their health goals.

Physical therapists are licensed healthcare professionals specializing in helping individuals recover from injuries and manage chronic conditions through physical therapy exercises.

Psychologists: Psychologists are healthcare professionals who specialize in mental health. They can provide counseling and therapy to help individuals manage mental health conditions and improve their well-being.

Conclusion

Working with a healthcare professional can provide a wide range of benefits for your health and well-being. Whether you're looking to manage a chronic condition, prevent disease, or improve your overall health, a healthcare professional can provide the expertise, guidance, and support you need to achieve your goals.

If you're interested in working with a healthcare professional, talk to your primary care provider or search for a healthcare professional in your area. You can unlock your full potential for optimal health with the proper support.

This page was left blank intentionally

Chapter Seven: Stay Motivated

He that conquer Mindset, can conquer anything

It can be challenging to lose weight, both bodily and psychologically. While most people only concentrate on the physical elements of weight reduction, it is crucial to understand the role that mindset plays in reaching your objectives. Your approach can significantly influence your success or failure with weight reduction.

Your mindset will significantly impact your weight reduction path. Your ideas and beliefs can influence your ability to maintain a healthy lifestyle and achieve your objectives about your capacity to lose weight, your sense of worth, and your motivations. This article will discuss the role of mentality in weight loss and offer advice on cultivating an optimistic mindset to help you on your weight loss path.

Why Mindset Is Important

Your attitude dramatically influences your ability to lose weight. It can influence your thoughts, feelings, and drive, which makes it a crucial element in deciding your success. Your attitude affects your ability to lose weight for the following reasons:

Your mindset influences your attitude

Your effectiveness in losing weight depends on how you feel about it. An unfavorable outlook can cause insecurity, despair, and a lack of drive. On the other hand, a positive outlook can assist you in maintaining your motivation, concentration, and optimism about your advancement.

Your mentality influences how you behave.

Your ideas and beliefs can immediately impact your behavior. You might be less likely to exert the effort necessary to reach your objectives if you think you can't lose weight or if it will be too difficult. On the other hand, you are more likely to take the necessary actions to succeed if you have faith in your ability to accomplish your objectives and are dedicated to making healthy decisions.

Your mindset impacts your emotions.

Your mindset and emotions can significantly impact how you behave and how you feel about your weight reduction path. Positive thoughts and beliefs can help you feel assured, empowered, and driven, whereas negative thoughts and beliefs can cause worry, sadness, and frustration.

Creating a Positive Mentality to Lose Weight

Given your newfound understanding of mindset's role in weight reduction, let's look at some techniques for cultivating an optimistic mindset to help you achieve your objectives.

Concentrate on the Procedure, Not Just the Result

While achieving your weight loss objectives is essential, it's equally important to concentrate on the procedure rather than just the result. Setting attainable objectives, acknowledging minor victories, and concentrating on daily routines and behaviors that promote long-term success are all aspects of a process-oriented mindset.

Adopt a growth mindset.

A growth mentality is a conviction that your potential can be realized through perseverance and diligent effort. Even when confronted with difficulties, adopting a development mentality can help you stay inspired and tenacious in your weight reduction path.

Use self-compassion.

Being kind to yourself as you lose weight can go a long way in easing the burden. Treating yourself with kindness, realizing that mistakes are a normal part of the process, and changing negative ideas into constructive ones are all components of practicing self-compassion.

Embrace the Supportive People in Your Life

Your social support network can significantly impact your weight reduction path. Look for friends, relatives, or a support group that can encourage, hold you accountable and motivate you. These people should share your objectives and beliefs.

Concentrate on Small-Scale Wins

Although weight is a crucial indicator of improvement, it is not the only one. You can maintain your motivation and confidence in your progress by concentrating on non-scale triumphs like increased vitality, better sleep, or improved mood.

Adopt a Mindful Eating Habit

Mindful eating is one of the best methods to cultivate a positive attitude toward weight reduction. To practice mindful eating, you should focus on your meal, enjoy each bite, and consume methodically. When you consume attentively, you become more conscious of the flavors and textures of your food, which enhances the enjoyment and increases feelings of fullness.

You can prevent overeating when you consume attentively because you are more conscious of your body's cues of hunger and satiety. Instead of eating out of genuine desire, many people do so for emotional or habitual reasons. You can learn to differentiate between physical and mental hunger by engaging in mindful eating practices, which will help you consume only when your body needs to be nourished.

Honor small victories

The importance of small victories in weight reduction is another crucial attitude component. Acknowledging and appreciating the little victories along the road is essential because losing weight is a journey. Take the time to recognize and appreciate these achievements, whether it's losing a few pounds, getting into a smaller size of apparel, or making healthier food choices.

You can stay motivated and on schedule for your weight reduction objectives by celebrating small victories. Additionally, it may help you develop the assurance and self-worth necessary for long-term achievement. To help reinforce good behavior, treat yourself to something you appreciate, like a new novel or a massage.

Find a Supportive Network

Having a support structure in place can be crucial because losing weight can be difficult. Having someone to share your path with, whether a buddy, a member of your family, or a support group, can help keep you accountable and inspired.

When you encounter difficulties or obstacles, your support network can inspire and assist you. They can share their knowledge and experiences with you, which can help you overcome challenges and maintain your weight reduction plans.

Engage in Self-Care

Self-care is a crucial component of attitude when trying to lose weight. Taking care of your bodily, emotional, and spiritual well-being is a form of self-care. It may involve having enough rest, working out frequently, and using stress-reduction strategies like deep breathing or meditation.

You are better equipped to handle the difficulties associated with weight reduction when you put self-care first. Additionally, you are more likely to have the drive and inspiration to make good decisions and adhere to your weight reduction strategy.

Be persistent and upbeat.

Finally, it's critical to maintain an optimistic outlook and persevere throughout your weight reduction process. It can be challenging to lose weight, and it's common to run into difficulties along the road. It's crucial to remember that these difficulties are only momentary and that you have the fortitude and resiliency necessary to get through them.

Pay attention to the good parts of your path, like how your health has improved and how your body has changed for the better. Maintain a positive outlook and regularly recall yourself of your objectives and the primary drivers behind starting your weight reduction adventure.

Tracking progress smartly

Any fitness or health quest must include tracking success. It lets you see your progress, keeps you responsible, and inspires you to keep trying. To monitor something successfully, though, or to know what to track, can be complicated. This piece will examine various strategies for tracking your development and managing your fitness and health objectives.

Make Specific Goals

Setting specific objectives is the first stage in monitoring your progress. Your objectives should be clear, quantifiable, doable, timely, and pertinent. (SMART). For instance, a SMART objective might be "I want to lose weight," instead of "I want to exercise three times a week and reduce my calorie intake to 1,500 calories per day."

Setting specific objectives lets you concentrate your efforts and precisely track your development. Additionally, it encourages and makes you feel successful when you achieve your objectives.

Implement a tracking tool.

Using a monitoring tool to keep track of your progress is the next step after deciding on your objectives. There are numerous options for monitoring instruments, including wearable technology, diaries, spreadsheets, and applications.

Pick a monitoring device that suits your needs and that you'll use regularly. MyFitnessPal, Fitbit, and Apple Health are a few of the well-liked monitoring programs.

Follow Important Metrics

It's crucial to monitor appropriate measures that support your objectives. If your objective is to drop weight, you should monitor your weight, body fat proportion, and waist size. You should monitor your resting heart rate, blood pressure, and cardio stamina to improve your cardiovascular health.

It's crucial to stay focused on the figures, though. Remember that measurements like weight are only one component of the overall image. Consider your general success toward your objectives, how you feel, how your clothes fit, and how you look.

Trends Over Time to Watch

It understands how you're doing and figuring out where you need to require better monitoring of your development over time. Examine the patterns in your data to see if you're regularly shedding weight if your resting heart rate is dropping, or if your stamina is increasing.

However, avoid getting too engrossed in daily variations. Weight and other measurements vary slightly from day to day due to water, menstruation, and tension. Instead, pay attention to the long-term pattern as a whole.

Honor small victories

Finally, remember to acknowledge and appreciate even the most minor victories. It can take a long time to lose weight or reach other health and fitness objectives, and losing motivation along the road is simple. Celebrating minor victories can boost your self-esteem and keep you inspired.

Small victories can be as simple as setting a new personal record while running, squeezing into a pair of previously unwearable pants, or receiving positive feedback about your development. Just keep in mind that any improvement is growth.

In conclusion, monitoring success is crucial to any exercise and health path. You can stay inspired and out of common traps by establishing clear goals, using a recording tool, watching pertinent data, observing patterns over time, and enjoying small victories. Always be kind to yourself and have faith in the process. You can reach your fitness and health objectives and realize your best potential with the appropriate attitude and resources.

Conclusion: Putting It All Together

In conclusion, achieving a healthy weight, increasing vitality, and balancing hormones are not tricky. Anyone can defeat obesity quickly with the correct information, strategy, and attitude and reach their desired physical characteristics and health objectives. Individuals can achieve durable and long-lasting results by concentrating on healthy routines like a balanced diet, regular exercise, and quality sleep and integrating techniques like mindfulness, monitoring progress, and getting support from healthcare experts.

It's crucial to remember that everyone's path to perfect health and well-being will be different, and there might be obstacles and difficulties along the way. However, people can stay on track toward their objectives and eventually experience greater well-being and energy by staying inspired, avoiding common mistakes, and enjoying even the tiniest triumphs.

So don't delay any longer if you're eager to take control of your health. Start today by making minor living adjustments, then progressively expand upon them. You can outsmart fat quickly and realize your maximum potential if you put effort into it, are persistent, and have an optimistic outlook.

Recap of the 7 secrets for fat burning

Many strategies and techniques are available for burning fat, but not all are equal. We've detailed 7 essential tips in this manual for beating fat quickly and reaching peak wellness. Now that we've reviewed those techniques let's examine how they can assist you in achieving your objectives.

Recognize Your Metabolism

You understand how your metabolism functions can help you make the most of your strategy because it significantly reduces fat. You can speed up your metabolism and support your body's natural fat-burning processes by emphasizing healthy behaviors like regular exercise, a balanced diet, and adequate sleep.

Your Hormone Balance

Balancing hormones like insulin and cortisol is essential for optimum health because they can affect weight loss. You can support your weight reduction efforts by reducing tension, consuming a balanced diet, and receiving enough sleep.

Nutritional Optimization

You can support your general health and reach your weight loss objectives by eating a well-balanced whole foods diet. Limit processed and refined foods in favor of nutrient-dense foods like fruits, veggies, whole cereals, and lean meats.

Increase your use of high-intensity interval training

HIIT, or high-intensity interval exercise, can help you lose weight and increase your fitness. You can increase your metabolism and the number of calories you expend by alternating between vigorous activity and rest.

Adopt a Mindful Eating Habit

By practicing mindful dining, you can learn to focus on your body's appetite and fullness cues and prevent overeating. You can establish a healthy connection with food and reach your weight reduction objectives by chewing your food thoroughly, eating slowly, and being aware of your body's signals.

Keep striving and stay away from common pitfalls.

Staying motivated and preventing typical pitfalls can be challenging, but doing so is crucial to your success. You can remain on schedule and reach your weight loss objectives by making reasonable goals, acknowledging little accomplishments, and getting help when necessary.

Track Your Progress Wisely

Monitoring your development can help you maintain motivation and make necessary corrections. To keep track of your success and spot areas where you need to make adjustments, use tools like a food journal, exercise log, or progress photos.

You can outwit fat quickly and accomplish your desired body and health goals by adding these 7 strategies to your weight reduction path. Everyone's path will be distinct, and it may take some time to discover the best strategy for you. But you can accomplish long-lasting and sustainable outcomes if you are committed, persistent, and optimistic.

This page was left blank intentionally

Creating a personalized weight loss plan

When you need help knowing where to begin or how to create a strategy that works for you, losing weight can be challenging and stressful. Even though there are numerous diets and weight reduction plans available, everyone's body and requirements are unique. Because of this, it's crucial to develop a customized weight-loss strategy that considers your unique objectives, way of life, and preferences.

You can follow the methods listed below to develop a weight reduction strategy that is effective for you:

Before beginning any weight reduction program, it's crucial to establish objectives that are both attainable and sustainable. Expecting to drop 20 pounds in a few weeks is unrealistic. Instead, strive for a weekly weight reduction of 1-2 pounds that is steady and gradual.

Evaluate your way of life: Examine your present way of living and note any areas where you can change it. Are you mostly idling during the day? Do you frequently ingest fast cuisine or consume a lot of processed food? By recognizing your current patterns, you can alter your lifestyle behaviors to support your weight reduction objectives.

Find out how many calories you need to drop weight: To lose weight, you must ingest fewer calories than you expend. To calculate your daily caloric requirements based on your age, gender, height, weight, and degree of exercise, use an internet tool.

Pick nutritious foods: Eat whole, nutrient-dense foods like fruits, veggies, lean protein, and whole carbohydrates. You can eat these items to stay full while giving your body the necessary vitamins and nutrients.

Make a food plan: A meal schedule can help you stay on track with your weight reduction goals. Think about planning your meals in preparation, bringing wholesome snacks with you, and reducing your consumption of high-calorie foods and beverages.

Include exercise: Any weight-loss strategy should include exercise. Start with minor adjustments, such as walking after supper or using the steps instead of the lift as you feel more at ease, and gradually up your fitness regimen.

Track your development: Keeping tabs on your development can help you remain inspired and make necessary changes. Use an app or notebook to keep track of your weight, measurements, and calorie consumption.

Recall that there is no one solution for weight reduction. You can position yourself for success and reach your goals healthy and lasting by developing a customized weight reduction strategy.